If found, please contact:

Name |

_____

Home |

_____

Mobile |

_____

Disclaimer

I am not a doctor, this book is about my personal migraine experiences and knowledge. It is for information only and does not provide medical advice. Please do not ignore professional medical advice or treatment, if needed.

After suffering for over two and a half decades, I have made some truly remarkable discoveries in the past few years that have literally changed my life. I now live almost completely migraine free – something I never thought possible.

I believe what I have learned could change others' lives too. I would never claim to be an 'expert' on migraines, however, I *do* claim to be an expert on *MY* migraines.

@Migraine7Steps – Twitter

When your diary at the end of this book is complete, the diary below is also available on Amazon.

Migraine Diary

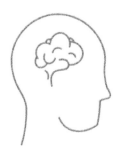

Record Symptoms

Identify Triggers

Take Control

Contents

Introduction   6

Migraine facts and stats   9

How it all started   10

Step 1: Understand the 'Contributory Factor'   11

Step 2: Identify and avoid triggers   13

Step 3: The Migraine Diary   21

Step 4: Eliminate fluoride   25

Step 5: Discover the (calcified) pineal gland   28

Step 6: Morning detox   32

Step 7: Stay hydrated   33

Bonus Step 1: Practise good health for the mind and body   35

Bonus Step 2: Have the right mindset   38

Conclusion   40

Acknowledgement   43

Migraine Annual Tracker   46

Migraine Event Tracker   47-94

Introduction

Welcome to the (not so) wonderful world of migraines. This book is written to provide information in simple, to the point, no nonsense language, largely avoiding complicated medical jargon.

Whether you are a migraine sufferer yourself, or you are reading this to help a friend, child or loved one, I truly believe this book will help you and I hope you will learn something you perhaps didn't know or had not considered. I'm in my late thirties now and I've been suffering with migraines since the age of 13.

I often wish I'd had access at that young age to the tips and suggestions in this book to help me. It's been a long journey.

One of the most frustrating things about migraines is that there are no two people exactly alike in the world when it comes to migraine symptoms and triggers. Yes, there are some commonalities, but it's impossible to find a solution to fit everyone.

I'm also sorry to inform you (if you don't already know), that unfortunately once a migraine sufferer... always a migraine sufferer. There is no 'cure' so to speak, but thankfully there are ways of hugely reducing, and almost completely eliminating, the amount and severity we have to endure. After doing what I have written about in this book for some years, I now no longer live my life wondering when the next migraine will hit. I basically took back control and, believe it or not, so can you.

The steps I follow take a daily effort to continue to live almost completely migraine free. Most of the steps can be implemented the moment you put the book down, and I whole-heartedly believe anyone, male or female, of any age group, suffering, from any kind of migraine, will benefit from this book. You really do get out what you put in.

It's true that migraines can be hereditary, as my father also suffers, however his symptoms and triggers are very different to mine, so it's a case of finding what works for you – I hope to help you with that. I learned long ago not to rely solely on medical experts. I became extremely fed up going to doctors (most of whom hadn't even experienced a migraine before) and straight away being prescribed medication that ultimately didn't work for me and came with many side effects.

I decided to take my situation into my own hands, take personal responsibility and recognise that I was the only one who actually cared about the suffering I was enduring. Please note: I do not talk about or recommend medication in this book as I do not take any at all.

So, if you are hoping for a 'quick fix' in the form of medication, then I'm afraid this book is not for you. During my time, I have tried all manner of medications to prevent and ease symptoms but nothing worked for me.

Many talk about migraines as inflammation in the brain, which is quite correct, and recommend NSAIDs (non-steroidal anti-inflammatory drugs) to help with this. However, I'm more keen on the idea of natural anti-inflammatories and alternatives as these do not have the many side effects of NSAIDs, so I found the advice to use medication unhelpful.

Personally, I would rather tackle the root cause of the issue than try to manage it with medication, which is like papering over the cracks. In a nutshell, prevention is truly **the** best cure!

I also won't be giving advice on vitamins or supplements. I do take some daily vitamins but, as advice on this is so contrasting, varies from person to person, and with the internet at your fingertips to research this, I will leave this information out of this book. I would highly recommend that you request an appointment with your doctor to do an overall health check and blood test, to find out if you have any allergies or deficiencies, and treat this accordingly specific to you.

The fact this book is a short read was very much intentional. I have read many books over the years and found them to be far too long, too complicated, full of medical jargon only doctors can understand and with no real substance in the end. I wanted the information to be quickly absorbed as, quite frankly, enough of our time has been lost due to migraines already.

I wrote this book as a migraine sufferer who, for over two and a half decades, suffered in silence. I grew tired of missing out on social events or other commitments to the invisible condition we suffer from. I've lost count of the many days in my life I have lost to debilitating migraine attacks and how many people I feel I have let down due to cancelling plans. I'm sure this will sound familiar to you.

Before I go any further I want to give you just a few facts and stats about migraines, which are worth knowing and can actually bring comfort that we are certainly not alone in our suffering.

Migraine facts and stats

Migraines are typically experienced in two forms; migraines with aura and migraines without aura.

There are of course other types, including chronic migraine, migraine with brainstem aura, menstrual migraine, abdominal migraine, hemiplegic migraine and vestibular migraine. For some people, even weather changes may cause imbalances in brain chemicals, including serotonin, which can contribute to a migraine.

About 10% of the UK population experiences migraines. Therefore, around 9 million people are suffering on a regular basis. Migraines can be acute (90%) or chronic (10%); with aura (10-30%) or without aura (70-90%). Migraines are the third most common disease in the world and have a global prevalence of 14.7%; that's around 1 in 7 people.

Being more prevalent than diabetes, epilepsy and asthma combined, the effect that migraines have on us shouldn't be underestimated.

They do not discriminate, migraines can happen to anyone. It's unfortunate for women that 1 in 5 will suffer as opposed to 1 in 15 men. They can begin at any age, although usually begin in the early years, and have been known to become less troublesome in later years.

Over 25 million work or school days are lost each year in the UK due to migraines.

For each one million of the UK population, 3,000 suffer migraine attacks. This equates to over 190,000 migraines every day!

How it all started

Being 13 years old and experiencing a debilitating migraine with aura for the first time was terrifying. To be introduced to the word migraine was a relief in the beginning, just to know I wasn't having a stroke or going blind. Little did I know that for the next 20+ years I would continue to suffer.

You may be wondering how often I had migraine attacks then compared to now. During my teens, I would typically have up to as many as half a dozen a week, to the point my teachers thought I was trying to get out of class as I was having them so frequently.

Until about five years ago, migraines literally ruled my life; in my teens and 20's, in particular, I always felt I was either experiencing the symptoms in the lead up to a migraine, the migraine itself or its after effects. I rarely felt 'normal' you could say.

I always felt I had this ticking migraine time bomb about to go off at any time in my head, so it was my first thought whenever I planned anything. "What if I have a migraine?" was always at the forefront of my mind – but not any more.

It is an ongoing process and requires day-to-day managing and being mindful of my activities, diet, health and wellbeing.

To go from almost half a dozen migraines a week to barely even one in a typical year is a great success and I truly feel I have full control over my migraines for the first time in my life.

Step 1: Understand the 'Contributory Factor'

Migraines are very complex but understanding the concept of how they work is actually quite simple – this is the first step.

We all have triggers that are entirely unique to us. As I mentioned in the introduction, there are no two people exactly alike in terms of their migraine symptoms and triggers. The 'contributory factor' term I created basically means that there are a number of individual triggers that contribute to our migraines. It's rarely just one specific trigger alone that causes a migraine and understanding this is paramount to taking back control.

To fully understand what I mean, it's like a pyramid of plastic drinking cups. Each one of those cups stacked up is a migraine trigger and whenever you identify a migraine trigger that affects you – eliminate it from your life. This means the pyramid of cups is smaller, has less chance of crashing down and resulting in you having a migraine. It may sound like I am over simplifying it but it really is that simple.

The only challenging things are 1. identifying your own specific triggers and 2. having the willpower to avoid these – just ask yourself, is this (trigger) worth contributing to me having a migraine. For me, nothing is worth it.

In the next step, I discuss the migraine triggers that I personally have identified, some or all of which may or may not also affect you. Then in step 3, I talk about the crucially important migraine diary, which explains exactly how I came to identify these.

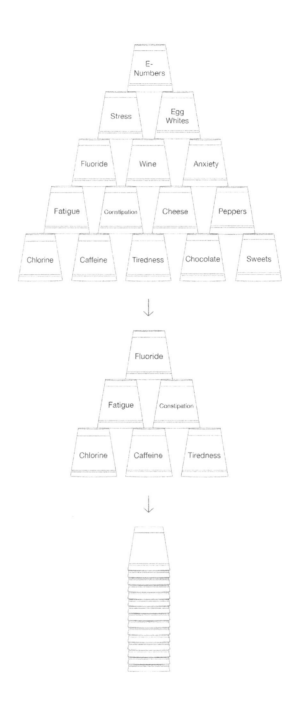

Step 2: Identify and avoid triggers

Before I go on to talk about the specific triggers I've identified, I wanted to talk a little about my symptoms. These will no doubt differ in some way to yours, but there may be some similarities. I have migraines with aura, which I would describe as beginning with seeing a small pin point dot that expands across most of my vision and goes off to either the left or right side. At times, it can also be likened to looking through a kaleidoscope and seeing flickering/flashing lights. With this, I can also experience headaches, confusion, fuzzy head, sensitivity to light, tingling nose and fingertips, nausea and sometimes affected speech.

Typically, the visual aura moves across to the left side of my vision. However, I have noticed that if it moves across to the right, which is very rare for me, I also have a pounding headache, something I don't often experience when the aura moves to the left. I have no explanation for this.

Telltale signs of a possible migraine coming can be very useful to identify and recognise. Usually, a migraine can start literally out of nowhere. Suddenly, in the blink of an eye, the pin point dot appears in my vision and that's it, I have to stop whatever I am doing and wait for the migraine to pass, which can take from one hour up to several hours.

In some of my worst migraine attacks, these have lasted on and off up to 24 hours, but this is rare for me. Signs that a migraine is possibly about to hit can include a tightness in my forehead, neck and jaw, also feeling irritable, frustrated or angry for no apparent reason, forgetfulness and also a low mood or feeling depressed. In contrast, an unexplained feeling of elation and a sudden burst of energy can also be a sign that a migraine is coming – but not always, of course.

Triggers

The crucial second step is recognising, and avoiding, your own specific triggers. I have dedicated steps in this book to fluoride and the (calcified) pineal gland, which have been two of the biggest connected revelations and have proven to be truly life changing, but first I will talk about other triggers I have identified:

- Chlorine – this being one of the chief causes of the calcified pineal gland (see step 5) was another of the big revelations I recognised from my migraine diary.

- Constipation – this can be a migraine trigger, due to the level of serotonin dropping in the intestines.

- Excessive lip biting, grinding teeth, chewing gum – really any activities that increase stress and strain on the jaw can result in it having to work harder and can contribute to a migraine attack. The temporo-mandibular joint (T.M.J. – the joint connecting your lower jaw and skull) may be worth asking your dentist or local chiropractor about. Symptoms of this are grinding your teeth, having difficulty opening your mouth fully, if your jaw locks when you open your mouth or if you hear a popping, clicking or grinding when you move your jaw. This is something that I had signs of so I currently do daily stretching exercises to keep my neck and jaw loose – they will be able to advise you on specific treatment for you.

- Excessive loud music from headphones – it's recognised that some who develop a headache or migraine from noise have an increase in their temporal pulse amplitude.

- Eye strain and being in dark or poor lighting conditions – having an eye test is recommended.

- Hunger and low blood sugar (hypoglycaemia) – it is crucial to have a filling breakfast (I have a large bowl of porridge with a teaspoon of flax seeds and chia seeds, one diced strawberry and ten or so blueberries with honey) and snack regularly, as this maintains a steady blood sugar and prevents hunger.

- Intense or heavy workout sessions – exercise is important for maintaining a healthy body and mind, however exercising in excess can have a negative effect on migraine sufferers. This could be due to reduced oxygen and fluid levels if you have not fuelled your body prior to working out.

- Poor posture – this results in tension build up in the neck, shoulders and upper back, which can contribute to migraines.

- Sitting in a poorly ventilated, stuffy, hot room or vehicle – this causes low oxygen while the good air is reduced in the space you are in. Your brain requires a lot of oxygen to function and, if it is starved of this, there is a higher risk of migraine. The solution to this is to always, if possible, have fresh air entering the space.

- Stress, worry and anxiety – when you are under stress, levels of certain molecules and hormones go up or down in some people – these changes can trigger a migraine.

- Strong smells, fumes and chemicals – migraine sufferers are extra sensitive to these due to increased activation of specific scent and pain receptors in the brain.

- Tiredness and lack of sleep; alternatively too much sleep and long lie ins are not recommended.

All of these, and more, can contribute to our migraines. There will of course be other commonly known triggers but these are the triggers I have currently identified that affect me. Over time, and with the help of my migraine diary, more will no doubt come to my attention.

The exact cause of migraines is largely unknown, but is thought to be the result of temporary changes in chemicals, blood vessels and nerves in the brain. It is absolutely crucial to have daily (natural) anti-inflammatories – I will go into this a little later and explain my method.

Flashing and flickering lights can also affect migraine sufferers, however, even though this is one of the most commonly known triggers, it is actually one of the smallest and least likely contributors – this is a fact that surprised me when I first heard it.

I can vouch for this as a photographer with a professional studio who uses strobe flash lighting. If you would like to view my photography please visit **andrewjshearer.co.uk** ...yes that was a shameless plug!

The following are dietary triggers I have identified for myself. They may or may not be relevant to you, but for me they include:

- Apple juice – 100% avoid as high in tannins and nitrates.

- Caffeine – some people claim this helps their migraines however I 100% avoid it as it actually affects the activity of a naturally occurring brain substance called adenosine and causes this to increase. As well as coffee, I avoid tea as this is also high in tannins, which is a common migraine trigger.

- Cheese, particularly aged cheeses – 100% avoid – I use a coconut oil substitute cheese.

- Chocolate – 100% avoid as it contains the amino acid tyramine – however, I can eat white chocolate from any 'free from' range.

- Corn – I avoid because it is very inflammatory and difficult to digest. It is also a common migraine trigger.

- Dairy – 100% avoid as I drink goat's milk and use dairy-free products. It's recommended to reduce dairy such as milk, low-fat milk, cheeses, margarine and products with milk additives. It's been recognised that over 70% of migraine sufferers became almost migraine free after the elimination of dairy.

- Egg whites – avoid if possible – as these include excessive amounts of glutamic acid, which is a top migraine trigger.

- Fizzy drinks – 100% avoid as many contain caffeine and/or the sweetener aspartame.

- Foods/beverages that contain aspartame (aspartame sweetener consists of the amino acids aspartic acid and phenylalanine). Also foods with phenylethylamine, tannins, nitrates and tyramine should be largely avoided, if possible. The flavour enhancer M.S.G. (monosodium glutamate) is also not recommended.

- Gluten – this is not exactly a recognised definitive migraine trigger, however many migraine sufferers do believe gluten may be a trigger for them. I went gluten free some years ago for an unrelated reason and haven't looked back.

- Grapes – 100% avoid as high in tyramine.

- Meat that has been aged, smoked, salted or has had tenderiser added can potentially be a trigger and should ideally be avoided.

- Nuts – 100% avoid at all costs, especially walnuts and pecans, which contain tyramine.

- Oranges – 100% avoid as high in tyramine.

- Salt – it's thought that salty processed foods may have harmful preservatives that could trigger migraines, as high levels of sodium can increase blood pressure. Conversely, if the migraine is due to an electrolyte imbalance caused by dehydration, adding a little salt and/or sugar to water could actually help. Personally, I try to have a low salt intake and actually use pink Himalayan salt as this is a natural and healthier alternative.

- Spicy/hot food – it's more likely chilli peppers than the spicy or hot food that will trigger a migraine as these react to certain pain receptors (called TRP receptors) in the brain, which lowers the threshold for developing a migraine.

- Sweets/candy – I choose to 100% avoid as they contain a variety of E-numbers, artificial sweeteners, flavourings, colourings and preservatives. Consuming a lot of sugar can cause hyperglycemia and lead to migraines. Alternatively, too little sugar hypoglycemia, mentioned earlier, can cause migraines.

- Wine – I avoid wine completely; red wine, in particular, should be avoided as it contains biogenic amines, which are problematic for the brain, and preservatives like sulphites. It also causes a very high rise in serotonin (5-HT) in the blood and, as it is made from grapes, also has a high tyramine content.

The following I find are acceptable in small doses but excessive consumption can contribute to a migraine attack:

- Alcohol – this is a diuretic – it acts on kidneys making people urinate more fluid than they are consuming, leading to dehydration, which can cause migraines. So, drinking to excess is ideally avoided but, as they say, "everything in moderation". Personally, I rarely drink but when I do, I find it helps to have a glass of water in between alcoholic drinks and, as mentioned, I avoid wine.

- Bananas – over-ripe bananas (which have increased tyramine content) are a trigger, however I find just-ripe bananas are fine. Bananas actually contain potassium, magnesium and B vitamins – all components that contribute to headache relief.

- Nightshade vegetables such as aubergines, potatoes, sweet potatoes, sweet/hot/chilli peppers and tomatoes contain neurotoxic alkaloids that can trigger a migraine and should ideally be avoided, however I personally find these acceptable in small amounts.

- Pineapple – containing tyramine, pineapple consumed in high amounts can cause migraines. However, in small amounts pineapple can act as a natural pain relief as it has the natural enzyme bromelain and boasts anti-inflammatory properties.

- Strawberries – in small amounts I find these acceptable but, like other fruits when they are over-ripe, tyramine content will increase so you should avoid consuming in large amounts.

As much as I've talked about foods that should be avoided, it's not all doom and gloom. Yes there are a number of foods and ingredients that ideally as migraine sufferers we should not consume, but there are many things we can enjoy.

It's a case of identifying for yourself what you can and can't have. This is where the migraine diary comes in...

Step 3: The Migraine Diary

This is a tip I remember someone giving me in my teens and I didn't listen to them – I wish I had. How on earth can we know what is causing the migraines we suffer if we don't have a record to look back on and notice patterns?

I will stress this again, it is vitally important to understand and recognise what your own individual triggers are. It is an absolutely crucial step in taking ownership of your migraines and how frequently you will suffer.

At the end of this book there is a short diary for you to start recording your migraines. I also published a larger diary (this is also available on Amazon) that you can use to continue your tracking once you have completed this book. I have used this for some years to record my migraine attacks and it has proven to be invaluable.

The diary contains the following information, which I add as soon after a migraine as possible:

- Date
- Time started, ended and duration
- Symptoms experienced
- Severity (1-9)
- Sleep
- Brief description of activities and any possible relevant triggers in the past 48 hours
- Breakfast, lunch, dinner, supper, snacks and water intake in the past 48 hours

The diary also has an annual tracker, which is very useful to see at a glance how many migraines have occurred throughout the year.

I would recommend filling in the diary for at least six months, but would highly recommend you keep it going for the rest of your life. We change as we get older and may recognise new symptoms and triggers.

Migraine Diary

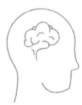

Record Symptoms

Identify Triggers

Take Control

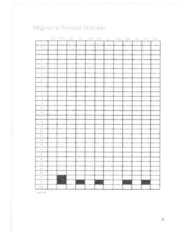

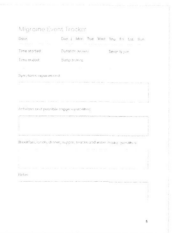

After six months, take your time to read through the diary and write down any patterns you notice. For example, I noticed that after every time I went to my local swimming pool I had a migraine that day or the day after, the culprit – chlorine. This is just one example, but I have recognised many of the triggers mentioned in step two by using this technique, particularly dietary ones.

After noticing a pattern, I would recommend eliminating the suspected trigger. If, however, the potential trigger is something you cannot find an alternative for and ideally would not like to give up, try re-entering it into your life and keep a close eye on your migraine diary to see if the same pattern develops around that trigger.

Should it become crystal clear and there is no doubt about a particular trigger, the decision is yours as to whether it's worth having a migraine or not. As I said, for me, nothing is worth it.

Step 4: Eliminate fluoride

I accidentally came across the link between fluoride and migraines some years ago without realising it at first. I had some (unrelated) tests done to identify any allergies and also if my body was lacking in any vitamins. I was told my body didn't react well to fluoride and it was recommended I eliminate my exposure to it – thankfully where I live here in Scotland, the water is not fluoridated, but I was using a fluoride toothpaste twice daily and had been all my life. I wasn't told anything about how and why it affects me, and at the time I didn't ask, but I cut out fluoride toothpaste from then on. During the next two years, I had only a couple of migraines! I didn't make the connection at first; I just thought maybe I was finally outgrowing them.

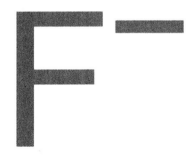

However, one day I ran out of my fluoride-free toothpaste and used my wife's (fluoride) toothpaste until mine arrived in the mail, as I ordered this online. In the space of seven days, I had five migraines!! More than double I'd had in the previous two years. Sat in my living room alone and somewhat depressed as I recovered from my fifth migraine that week, I thought to myself "what have I changed in the past week to make me have so many migraines?!". I realised the only thing I had done differently was to go back to using a fluoride toothpaste and then it hit me – I remembered being told previously about my body not reacting well to fluoride – never before have I had such a lightbulb moment.

I immediately googled the words 'fluoride and migraine' and found other people who had also recognised that when they consumed fluoride – whether it be during their time living in a country where the water is fluoridated and/or when using a fluoride toothpaste – they noticed their migraines were significantly worse. I sat in shock at what I had just discovered.

Immediately, I went back to my fluoride-free toothpaste and I didn't have another migraine for several months until I visited the dentist where they did a scale and polish. Unbeknown to me, this procedure includes the application of a strong fluoride-based paste and, as soon as it was applied, I tasted it in my mouth and realised what it was. My heart sank.

I felt off for the rest of that day and then early the very next day had a horrendous migraine. As it is a particularly strong fluoride paste used in dentistry for this treatment, I also felt unwell for two or three days afterwards and then had a cluster of migraines. I believe this was the strong substance working its way out of my system as I did not have another migraine until nearly a year later.

I cannot stress enough just how ill I felt during this week. I felt a weakness and tingling down my left side, a definite reduction to reaction times and functioning normally. My wife even noticed I was almost appearing in slow motion as I went about certain tasks, not able to grasp even the simplest of instructions.

I am convinced this is too much to be coincidental. I researched the connection between fluoride and migraines further and there is a recognised link, but it is very much not commonly known.

You may have read about my experience with fluoride and be quizzically thinking, "but I use fluoridated toothpaste (and/or water) every day... and I don't get a migraine every day". I understand this way of thinking but once you understand the contributory factor 'pyramid' it starts to make sense. Simply put, having fluoride in our body greatly increases the likelihood of other triggers we are exposed to resulting in migraine attacks. Compared to how our brain can fend off other potential triggers when we do not have the toxic fluoride substance coursing through our central nervous system.

I would implore you to try going fluoride free for at least a few months (it takes around 2-4 weeks to leave your system) and see if it makes a difference to you – this is the fourth step. After all, it takes little effort to buy one kind of toothpaste over another so you have nothing to lose and everything to gain. I personally use Kingfisher (mint) fluoride-free toothpaste, available on Amazon, containing no artificial sweeteners, flavourings, colourings or preservatives. If you live in fluoridated water areas (you can find this out online), buying a suitable water filter or consuming only bottled water is a simple solution.

To sum up, fluoride in migraine sufferers creates excess unwanted electrical activity in the brain and makes us more susceptible to migraine attacks. However, it also has many other negative effects on the brain and body, which you can research further online. But, a particularly relevant one that is important to us migraine sufferers is how it impacts on sleep quality by calcifying the pineal gland and lowering melatonin and serotonin levels – I'll talk about these in the next step as both are produced by the pineal gland. This was another major revelation, which is very much also connected to fluoride.

Step 5: Discover the (calcified) pineal gland

I came across the pineal gland purely by chance when researching the negative effects fluoride has on us. It is also known as the 'pineal body' and is a small pea-sized endocrine gland. It is located on the back portion of the third cerebral ventricle of the brain and is sometimes referred to as the 'third eye'.

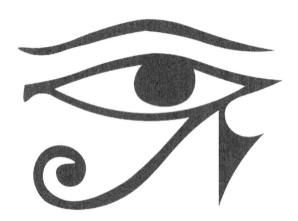

It produces and regulates melatonin, which is known for modulating our sleeping patterns in both circadian and seasonal cycles and is what we need to feel tired. If the pineal gland is calcified (something which fluoride, along with chlorine and synthetic calcium are the chief causes of), it can result in various medical conditions including insomnia and, more importantly to us, migraine attacks, which is not commonly known. Melatonin (and serotonin, which is also produced by the pineal gland – I'll talk about this in a moment) are quite the opposite to each other and they perform very different roles, but they need to work together in harmony to keep the body balanced.

Melatonin is a neurotransmitter-like substance. It is produced in the pineal gland when you are in dark surroundings. The melatonin winds the body down to prepare for sleep. To trick the brain into getting into that state is quite easy to do. Dim the lights and avoid the blue light emitted from televisions, devices and computers an hour or so before bed to increase melatonin levels.

Melatonin

Ideally, devices should be kept outside the bedroom as not only does having these there increase the chance of being awakened in the night, but it also increases the temptation to check your phone when you should be sleeping. If you're thinking "but it's my alarm clock", as the wise Simon Sinek said "buy an alarm clock!"

The connection between the pineal gland, fluoride and migraine should not be underestimated. It is extremely important to have a good sleep routine and ideally, if possible, go to sleep and wake up at the same time each day. Also avoid long lie-ins to keep a good circadian rhythm.

A couple of bonus tips regarding regulating sleeping patterns – for example, did you know a bowl of fresh mango an hour before bed helps to prevent insomnia and can promote a better night's sleep? In fact, in some countries mangoes are used as a natural sleep aid, preferred over sleep medications.

I also count back from 1,000 and picture the numbers in my mind each night to drift off to sleep – by the time I get down to around 950 I'm just about out for the count. I also suffer with tinnitus (constant ringing in ears) so if this method can help me to get to sleep it can help anyone!

Getting back to the pineal gland. Serotonin, which I mentioned earlier, is a neurotransmitter. This is a hormone that increases relaxation and positivity. It also helps us to feel more energised and generally happy. While melatonin is about the night, darkness and sleep, serotonin is about the morning, brightness and being awake. You can boost these levels by letting in the morning sunlight and fresh air.

Serotonin

A low level of serotonin in the brain can be a cause of migraines. People who suffer from weather-related migraines, due to imbalances in brain chemicals, are affected by low serotonin.

Often people with weather-related migraines feel there is nothing they can do about these. I appreciate there is nothing you can do about the weather itself, however there is actually much you can do to help your body and brain 'react' to those seasonal changes, i.e. keeping well hydrated and maintaining good sleep can only help. It is also important to decalcify the pineal gland, as doing this helps this type of migraine by increasing the amount of serotonin it produces.

Low levels of serotonin in the brain has also been linked to depression, which may explain why, when we suffer migraines, we also feel so low. Yes, we are fed up with migraines, how this impacts on our lives and makes us feel depressed, but it's also due to the calcified pineal gland and it actually being unable to produce that vital serotonin we need to feel happy and upbeat. I can tell you from personal experience that since I started decalcifying my pineal gland daily and living migraine free, I have never felt happier and more positive about the future.

This could be a 200-page book and still not fully cover the pineal gland, so I would encourage you to read up on this further online. But the takeaway to remember is that a calcified pineal gland in us migraine sufferers is a recipe for disaster.

I will explain in the next step how I daily decalcify this by having a morning detox drink with three essential key ingredients, which are crucial for migraine sufferers to consume.

Step 6: Morning detox

As mentioned, I decalcify the pineal gland every day first thing in the morning. I do this by having a big mug of warm/hot water with a tablespoon of fresh lemon juice, a tablespoon of Bragg's organic raw apple cider vinegar and the tip of a teaspoon of turmeric. Daily intake of turmeric is essential due to its incredible antioxidant and anti-inflammatory properties. I feel I should warn you the drink is not exactly pleasant to drink, quite frankly, it tastes horrible! However, very few 'medicines' or remedies ever do, if any. It takes seconds to drink and is definitely worth it, I assure you.

I first came across this around the beginning of my first two years living fluoride-free. My aim at the time was to have a morning detox drink to help my immune system, for an unrelated reason. Little did I know I was unknowingly decalcifying the pineal gland at the same time. As I later found out, from researching fluoride and the pineal gland, one of the best ways to actually decalcify the pineal gland is to have daily fresh lemon juice in warm/hot water.

As a result of further reading, I then came across the benefits of also adding Bragg's raw apple cider vinegar and turmeric to this. I haven't looked back since. I truly believe this is a natural miracle for migraine sufferers as I have encouraged others to try it for themselves and they are also amazed at the impact it has had on their lives, combined with following the other steps in this book.

This revelation really did bring it all together and I talk a bit more about this in the conclusion of this book.

Step 7: Stay hydrated

The seventh step – drink water! Increased water intake improves migraine symptoms by reducing the severity and frequency of these. I consume around two litres (equal to around 8 glasses) of water each day. I use a Super Sparrow one-litre stainless steel water bottle. Sufficient water intake is essential as being dehydrated throws off melatonin and serotonin balances.

$$H_2O$$

I previously used water filters but don't anymore. (There is a lot of contrasting information online as to whether it is necessary to filter your water or not.)

There are pros and cons of both drinking filtered and non-filtered water and I must say I've noticed no difference, apart from the money saved on not having to buy expensive water filter cartridges regularly – so it's up to you whether you do this or not, the main thing is to stay hydrated.

There are several reasons I keep my water at room temperature and why I avoid chilled water straight from the fridge. Cold water restricts digestion and hinders the natural process of absorbing nutrients. It can also result in sore throats and a stuffy nose through the buildup of excess mucus. It could also decrease heart rate as the low temperature of the water stimulates the heart rate to drop.

A bonus tip I learned from experience is to consume the water as early as you can in the day and ideally finish by late afternoon. Drinking water in the evening will increase the chance of waking up in the night needing to go to the loo, and with disturbed/lack of sleep being a trigger, this is counterproductive.

It's not entirely clear why dehydration triggers a migraine but, as a third of migraine sufferers, including myself, claim dehydration is a top trigger, it shouldn't be ignored. Afterall, human bodies are around 60% water so consuming it is essential.

Dehydration is very much an avoidable migraine trigger. The next step is a bonus about good health for the mind and body.

Bonus Step 1: Practise good health for the mind and body

Exercise can naturally boost your mood and feeling of wellbeing. This decreases our sensitivity to pain because exercise releases endorphins in the brain, reduces stress, stimulates the body to release natural anti-depressant chemicals called enkephalins and helps us to sleep well at night. I try to avoid overly strenuous or competitive exercising and I try to focus more on cardio and a variety of stretches each morning to keep my body, and neck in particular, loose.

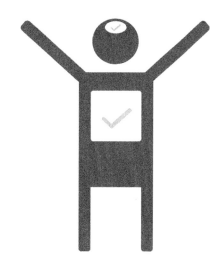

A typical morning exercise routine for me is to do various stretches and do a quick warm up, then row several miles on my rowing machine, a little weight training, before more stretches to cool down. It's a case of finding what works for you but generally it's recommended to do at least 30 minutes of exercise 3-4 times per week. I also try to walk when possible. It's worth mentioning it is important to have rest days to let your body recover.

Please remember, motion is lotion! This goes for the mind and body.

Something that is also worth including in your daily routine for your good health and reducing migraines is to meditate – please don't be put off by this suggestion. For many, when they hear the word meditation, they picture someone sitting with their legs crossed on the floor with their hands upturned on their knees making "ummmmmm" sounds!

Meditation for me is simply sitting on a seat with good posture, eyes closed, counting my breaths in and out for five minutes, and trying to clear my mind of all thoughts, stresses and worries. This is something that can be done at any time of day, when required. It's well known that mind-body techniques like meditation can relieve migraine and headaches by alleviating underlying stress.

Other useful ways to relieve stress and relax, which all contribute to preventing migraine attacks, are to take a warm bath, listen to some soothing music, receive a massage or read a good book, to name just a few.

Good health, of course, is also about diet and this plays a major part. In an ideal world, as migraine sufferers we should only consume natural produce with no artificial ingredients and regular (natural) anti-inflammatories.

Smoothies can be a fantastic way to consume fruit and veg that act as anti-inflammatories and there are endless recipes online to try. Green smoothies that contain green leafy vegetables, such as spinach and kale, are a great detox. Fruit smoothies containing, for example, cherries, watermelon, strawberries, pineapple and blueberries are also great anti-inflammatories.

With every smoothie drink I make, I add a teaspoon of flax seeds and chia seeds. Flax seeds are loaded with nutrients, improve cholesterol, lower blood pressure and are also high in omega 3, while chia seeds are loaded with antioxidants and are also high in omega 3.

Gut health is extremely important as a troubled intestine can send signals to the brain, and vice versa. Prebiotic foods that stimulate the healthy bacteria in the gut are recommended, such as a number of fruits and vegetables, legumes and grains.

Related to gut health, or more to the point *poor* gut health, is constipation – which can be a migraine trigger, due to the level of serotonin (which I spoke about earlier) dropping in the intestines.

As tempting as it is to eat fast food, junk food, processed food, sweets and drink to excess, if you fill the body with healthy natural goodness it can only respond by giving you good health in return. It really comes down to willpower, as I mentioned back in step one.

Mental health, of course, should not be overlooked as part of our health and wellbeing. Should you need some help there are several migraine trusts and associations you can contact for support. Related to migraines I would mainly recommend the following:

www.migrainetrust.org
www.nationalmigrainecentre.org.uk

(Also, please visit these websites for more facts and stats on migraines, some of which are included on page 9)

I would also highly recommend the fantastic **www.nhs.uk** here in the U.K. for support as they list a number of mental health charities and organisations.

Bonus Step 2: Have the right mindset

Generally there are two kinds of mindset:

- The fixed mindset – people who believe that qualities are fixed, inborn and unchangeable.
- The growth mindset – people who believe abilities can be developed and strengthened by commitment and hard work.

As human beings, when we lose something what are we programmed to do? To try to find it. This is why many people when trying to lose weight, for example, find it so difficult as they focus on what they have lost, i.e. junk food, being lazy and comfortable, as opposed to focusing on what they will *gain*, i.e. more energy, a healthier, longer life and the body they aspire to achieve.

This is applicable to our situation. Rather than focusing on what (triggers) we are losing from our lives and how much we are missing out on, we must focus on what we will gain, i.e. living migraine free and all the benefits in life that come with this.

If, like many others, you have the best intentions, but, after a while, things start to slip or maybe the enthusiasm starts to wane, then try using a daily checklist to keep yourself motivated.

This has been vital for me as I use a desk calendar that has space each day to write, with some simple checkboxes to tick, such as:

- ❏ 0600 wake up, and get up!
- ❏ Detox drink
- ❏ Motivational video/book
- ❏ Stretches routine

- ❏ Rowing/weights
- ❏ Mid-morning smoothie
- ❏ 2ltr water
- ❏ 2230 bed

The importance of ticking items on a checklist shouldn't be underestimated as this triggers dopamine in the brain, which is connected to feelings of pleasure and motivation.

You may wonder how long should you do this for – they say it takes around 66 days to form a habit. Previously, after a couple of months of doing a checklist I made the mistake of stopping this, thinking that as I had formed this habit, I didn't need to continue. I slowly started to slip back into my old routine.

Thankfully, I realised my mistake and corrected this by starting a new daily checklist and I haven't looked back since – I don't plan to stop doing it.

It's a case of doing what works for you. You may choose to do as I do or you may want to download an app or even use your phone calendar to pop up reminders each day to keep you on track.

Personally, I like ticking the checklist off and visibly seeing how many days I have achieved this as it really does give a boost of dopamine and a real sense of self-satisfaction.

In other words, adopt the right mindset and take control. Own the day, don't let it own you!

Conclusion

I want to make clear, I am not saying you will *never* experience another migraine again if you follow the steps in this book. We will still get a migraine at some point in our lives, when contributory factors and triggers that are beyond our control affect us. However, I hope your life will change for the better as much as mine has. There really is always hope, even though it may not feel like it sometimes.

Coming to terms with the fact we are migraine sufferers is one of the most important stages of taking ownership of our situation. For years when I was younger, I refused to even contemplate the idea of researching and learning about migraines, as I was in denial about the fact that I was largely responsible for the amount and severity of the migraines I had to endure. The last thing I wanted to do when I didn't have a migraine was to spend time reading about them! Now, with experience and hindsight, I now see I had it all wrong.

It may come as a surprise to some, but you really *are* responsible for the frequency and severity of the migraines you are having. I know that may be hard to swallow as it's easy to think it's just the hand we've been dealt and there is nothing much we can do about it. But, accepting personal responsibility and taking accountability is a crucial step to conquer. It truly is largely in our hands.

Many, myself included before I decided to take control, put little to no effort into tackling the root cause of migraines. I used to do all the wrong things, go about it all the wrong way and did absolutely nothing to help myself or my situation, and I wondered why I got so many migraines. Looking back now it's easy to see where I went wrong but without the knowledge I have today I realise I was just uneducated and so overwhelmed by the situation I didn't know which way to turn and what to do. I hope whatever age you are, you will know it's never too late to make a change and to start living migraine free.

By following the steps in this book, you can take back control, and you will also hopefully, one day soon, be able to live your life without the fear of when the next migraine will strike.

I made some of the discoveries in this book purely by chance and they have changed my life. For example, it was completely accidental that I discovered fluoride triggered migraines. Around this time I was researching ways I could try and improve my immune system, for an unrelated reason, and came across the tip to have the morning detox drink I talked about earlier – little did I know I was also decalcifying the pineal gland, something I only learned about when researching the effect fluoride has on us in relation to migraines.

With the help of my migraine diary, I discovered that chlorine was a top migraine trigger – which I later discovered was also one of the main causes of a calcified pineal gland.

As well as this, I increased my water intake to two litres a day, not realising at that time the incredible impact being hydrated has on the frequency of migraine attacks and pineal gland function. There have been a lot of coincidences that in the end were actually all connected, and I really believe if anyone follows the steps in this book it cannot fail to have a positive result.

Finally, I want to sum up in a nutshell the key takeaways from this book.

- Avoid fluoride, chlorine and commercial calcium supplements
- Complete a migraine diary after every attack, note possible triggers and avoid them!
- Learn about the pineal gland and decalcify this daily by having the morning detox drink
- Keep well hydrated with water and aim to consume around two litres daily
- Improve sleep pattern and quality, avoid those tempting lie-ins
- Exercise regularly and practise good health/diet for the mind and body
- Have a growth mindset, focus on what you have to gain and tick off that checklist!

I would like to thank you very much for purchasing this book. I would appreciate it if you would please leave feedback on Amazon and even let me know in your review how it has helped you.

Please share the Amazon link to this book and the diary with anyone you know who suffers with migraines, as these may be of help to them too.

There is also a Twitter page for this book @Migraine7Steps – please give me a follow and, if you want to ask any questions, feel free to contact me.

All the very best of luck to you ...from one migraineur to another,

- Andrew J Shearer

Acknowledgement

Writing this book has been the result of hearing others in conversation mention suffering with migraines and I have been intrigued by their reaction when they hear what I have learned, and the impact this has had on my situation. They either have one of two responses. One being of fascination and keen to try my steps for themselves. The other reaction is a more skeptical one as they fail to open their mind to the possibilities and realise they could actually take control.

So, to the people with both reactions at opposite ends of the scale I thank you, as I most likely wouldn't have thought of writing this book otherwise.

I would like to thank the woman (you know who you are Vera) who first noticed my body did not react well to fluoride. This, along with the revelations that came because of this information, changed my life in a way I could not have ever predicted.

Also, a special thank you to the woman in my life, Louise, who has been there for the past 14 years and counting, to offer her continued love and support ❤

Migraine Diary

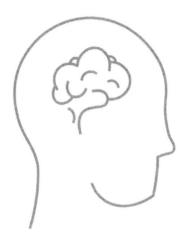

Record Symptoms

Identify Triggers

Take Control

Migraine Annual Tracker

	Jan	Feb	Mar	Apr	May	Jun	Jul	Aug	Sep	Oct	Nov	Dec
1												
2												
3												
4												
5												
6												
7												
8												
9												
10												
11												
12												
13												
14												
15												
16												
17												
18												
19												
20												
21												
22												
23												
24												
25												
26												
27												
28												
29		*										
30		■										
31		■		■		■			■		■	
Total												

* Leap year

Migraine Event Tracker

Date: Day | Mon   Tue   Wed   Thu   Fri   Sat   Sun

Time started: Duration (hr/min):   Severity (1-9):

Time ended: Sleep (hr/min):

Symptoms experienced

Activities and possible triggers (past 48hrs)

Breakfast, lunch, dinner, supper, snacks and water intake (past 48hrs)

Notes

Migraine Event Tracker

Date: Day | Mon Tue Wed Thu Fri Sat Sun

Time started: Duration (hr/min):   Severity (1-9):

Time ended: Sleep (hr/min):

Symptoms experienced

Activities and possible triggers (past 48hrs)

Breakfast, lunch, dinner, supper, snacks and water intake (past 48hrs)

Notes

Migraine Event Tracker

Date: Day | Mon   Tue   Wed   Thu   Fri   Sat   Sun

Time started: Duration (hr/min):   Severity (1-9):

Time ended: Sleep (hr/min):

Symptoms experienced

Activities and possible triggers (past 48hrs)

Breakfast, lunch, dinner, supper, snacks and water intake (past 48hrs)

Notes

Migraine Event Tracker

Date: Day | Mon Tue Wed Thu Fri Sat Sun

Time started: Duration (hr/min):   Severity (1-9):

Time ended: Sleep (hr/min):

Symptoms experienced

Activities and possible triggers (past 48hrs)

Breakfast, lunch, dinner, supper, snacks and water intake (past 48hrs)

Notes

Migraine Event Tracker

Date: Day | Mon   Tue   Wed   Thu   Fri   Sat   Sun

Time started: Duration (hr/min):   Severity (1-9):

Time ended: Sleep (hr/min):

Symptoms experienced

Activities and possible triggers (past 48hrs)

Breakfast, lunch, dinner, supper, snacks and water intake (past 48hrs)

Notes

Migraine Event Tracker

Date: Day | Mon   Tue   Wed   Thu   Fri   Sat   Sun

Time started: Duration (hr/min):   Severity (1-9):

Time ended: Sleep (hr/min):

Symptoms experienced

Activities and possible triggers (past 48hrs)

Breakfast, lunch, dinner, supper, snacks and water intake (past 48hrs)

Notes

Migraine Event Tracker

Date: Day | Mon   Tue   Wed   Thu   Fri   Sat   Sun

Time started: Duration (hr/min):   Severity (1-9):

Time ended: Sleep (hr/min):

Symptoms experienced

Activities and possible triggers (past 48hrs)

Breakfast, lunch, dinner, supper, snacks and water intake (past 48hrs)

Notes

Migraine Event Tracker

Date: Day | Mon   Tue   Wed   Thu   Fri   Sat   Sun

Time started: Duration (hr/min):   Severity (1-9):

Time ended: Sleep (hr/min):

Symptoms experienced

Activities and possible triggers (past 48hrs)

Breakfast, lunch, dinner, supper, snacks and water intake (past 48hrs)

Notes

Migraine Event Tracker

Date: Day | Mon   Tue   Wed   Thu   Fri   Sat   Sun

Time started: Duration (hr/min):   Severity (1-9):

Time ended: Sleep (hr/min):

Symptoms experienced

Activities and possible triggers (past 48hrs)

Breakfast, lunch, dinner, supper, snacks and water intake (past 48hrs)

Notes

Migraine Event Tracker

Date: Day | Mon   Tue   Wed   Thu   Fri   Sat   Sun

Time started: Duration (hr/min):   Severity (1-9):

Time ended: Sleep (hr/min):

Symptoms experienced

Activities and possible triggers (past 48hrs)

Breakfast, lunch, dinner, supper, snacks and water intake (past 48hrs)

Notes

Migraine Event Tracker

Date: Day | Mon   Tue   Wed   Thu   Fri   Sat   Sun

Time started: Duration (hr/min):   Severity (1-9):

Time ended: Sleep (hr/min):

Symptoms experienced

Activities and possible triggers (past 48hrs)

Breakfast, lunch, dinner, supper, snacks and water intake (past 48hrs)

Notes

Migraine Event Tracker

Date: _____   Day | Mon   Tue   Wed   Thu   Fri   Sat   Sun

Time started: _____   Duration (hr/min): _____   Severity (1-9): _____

Time ended: _____   Sleep (hr/min): _____

Symptoms experienced

[   ]

Activities and possible triggers (past 48hrs)

[   ]

Breakfast, lunch, dinner, supper, snacks and water intake (past 48hrs)

[   ]

Notes

[   ]

Migraine Event Tracker

Date: Day | Mon   Tue   Wed   Thu   Fri   Sat   Sun

Time started: Duration (hr/min):   Severity (1-9):

Time ended: Sleep (hr/min):

Symptoms experienced

Activities and possible triggers (past 48hrs)

Breakfast, lunch, dinner, supper, snacks and water intake (past 48hrs)

Notes

Migraine Event Tracker

Date: Day | Mon Tue Wed Thu Fri Sat Sun

Time started: Duration (hr/min): Severity (1-9):

Time ended: Sleep (hr/min):

Symptoms experienced

Activities and possible triggers (past 48hrs)

Breakfast, lunch, dinner, supper, snacks and water intake (past 48hrs)

Notes

Migraine Event Tracker

Date: Day | Mon   Tue   Wed   Thu   Fri   Sat   Sun

Time started: Duration (hr/min):   Severity (1-9):

Time ended: Sleep (hr/min):

Symptoms experienced

```



```

Activities and possible triggers (past 48hrs)

```



```

Breakfast, lunch, dinner, supper, snacks and water intake (past 48hrs)

```



```

Notes

```



```

Migraine Event Tracker

Date: Day | Mon   Tue   Wed   Thu   Fri   Sat   Sun

Time started: Duration (hr/min):   Severity (1-9):

Time ended: Sleep (hr/min):

Symptoms experienced

Activities and possible triggers (past 48hrs)

Breakfast, lunch, dinner, supper, snacks and water intake (past 48hrs)

Notes

Migraine Event Tracker

Date: Day | Mon   Tue   Wed   Thu   Fri   Sat   Sun

Time started: Duration (hr/min):   Severity (1-9):

Time ended: Sleep (hr/min):

Symptoms experienced

Activities and possible triggers (past 48hrs)

Breakfast, lunch, dinner, supper, snacks and water intake (past 48hrs)

Notes

Migraine Event Tracker

Date: Day | Mon   Tue   Wed   Thu   Fri   Sat   Sun

Time started: Duration (hr/min):   Severity (1-9):

Time ended: Sleep (hr/min):

Symptoms experienced

Activities and possible triggers (past 48hrs)

Breakfast, lunch, dinner, supper, snacks and water intake (past 48hrs)

Notes

Migraine Event Tracker

Date: Day | Mon   Tue   Wed   Thu   Fri   Sat   Sun

Time started: Duration (hr/min):   Severity (1-9):

Time ended: Sleep (hr/min):

Symptoms experienced

Activities and possible triggers (past 48hrs)

Breakfast, lunch, dinner, supper, snacks and water intake (past 48hrs)

Notes

Migraine Event Tracker

Date: Day | Mon   Tue   Wed   Thu   Fri   Sat   Sun

Time started: Duration (hr/min):   Severity (1-9):

Time ended: Sleep (hr/min):

Symptoms experienced

Activities and possible triggers (past 48hrs)

Breakfast, lunch, dinner, supper, snacks and water intake (past 48hrs)

Notes

Migraine Event Tracker

Date: Day | Mon   Tue   Wed   Thu   Fri   Sat   Sun

Time started: Duration (hr/min):   Severity (1-9):

Time ended: Sleep (hr/min):

Symptoms experienced

Activities and possible triggers (past 48hrs)

Breakfast, lunch, dinner, supper, snacks and water intake (past 48hrs)

Notes

Migraine Event Tracker

Date: Day | Mon   Tue   Wed   Thu   Fri   Sat   Sun

Time started: Duration (hr/min):   Severity (1-9):

Time ended: Sleep (hr/min):

Symptoms experienced

Activities and possible triggers (past 48hrs)

Breakfast, lunch, dinner, supper, snacks and water intake (past 48hrs)

Notes

Migraine Event Tracker

Date: _____ Day | Mon Tue Wed Thu Fri Sat Sun

Time started: _____ Duration (hr/min): _____ Severity (1-9): _____

Time ended: _____ Sleep (hr/min): _____

Symptoms experienced

Activities and possible triggers (past 48hrs)

Breakfast, lunch, dinner, supper, snacks and water intake (past 48hrs)

Notes

Migraine Event Tracker

Date: _____ Day | Mon Tue Wed Thu Fri Sat Sun

Time started: _____ Duration (hr/min): _____ Severity (1-9): _____

Time ended: _____ Sleep (hr/min): _____

Symptoms experienced

```
|                                                                      |
|                                                                      |
|                                                                      |
|                                                                      |
```

Activities and possible triggers (past 48hrs)

```
|                                                                      |
|                                                                      |
|                                                                      |
|                                                                      |
```

Breakfast, lunch, dinner, supper, snacks and water intake (past 48hrs)

```
|                                                                      |
|                                                                      |
|                                                                      |
|                                                                      |
```

Notes

```
|                                                                      |
|                                                                      |
|                                                                      |
|                                                                      |
```

Migraine Event Tracker

Date: _____ Day | Mon Tue Wed Thu Fri Sat Sun

Time started: _____ Duration (hr/min): _____ Severity (1-9): _____

Time ended: _____ Sleep (hr/min): _____

Symptoms experienced

Activities and possible triggers (past 48hrs)

Breakfast, lunch, dinner, supper, snacks and water intake (past 48hrs)

Notes

Migraine Event Tracker

Date: Day | Mon   Tue   Wed   Thu   Fri   Sat   Sun

Time started: Duration (hr/min):   Severity (1-9):

Time ended: Sleep (hr/min):

Symptoms experienced

```
┌─────────────────────────────────────────────────────────────────────┐
│                                                                       │
│                                                                       │
│                                                                       │
│                                                                       │
└─────────────────────────────────────────────────────────────────────┘
```

Activities and possible triggers (past 48hrs)

```
┌─────────────────────────────────────────────────────────────────────┐
│                                                                       │
│                                                                       │
│                                                                       │
│                                                                       │
└─────────────────────────────────────────────────────────────────────┘
```

Breakfast, lunch, dinner, supper, snacks and water intake (past 48hrs)

```
┌─────────────────────────────────────────────────────────────────────┐
│                                                                       │
│                                                                       │
│                                                                       │
│                                                                       │
└─────────────────────────────────────────────────────────────────────┘
```

Notes

```
┌─────────────────────────────────────────────────────────────────────┐
│                                                                       │
│                                                                       │
│                                                                       │
└─────────────────────────────────────────────────────────────────────┘
```

Migraine Event Tracker

Date: Day | Mon Tue Wed Thu Fri Sat Sun

Time started: Duration (hr/min): Severity (1-9):

Time ended: Sleep (hr/min):

Symptoms experienced

Activities and possible triggers (past 48hrs)

Breakfast, lunch, dinner, supper, snacks and water intake (past 48hrs)

Notes

Migraine Event Tracker

Date: Day | Mon Tue Wed Thu Fri Sat Sun

Time started: Duration (hr/min):   Severity (1-9):

Time ended: Sleep (hr/min):

Symptoms experienced

Activities and possible triggers (past 48hrs)

Breakfast, lunch, dinner, supper, snacks and water intake (past 48hrs)

Notes

Migraine Event Tracker

Date: Day | Mon   Tue   Wed   Thu   Fri   Sat   Sun

Time started: Duration (hr/min):   Severity (1-9):

Time ended: Sleep (hr/min):

Symptoms experienced

Activities and possible triggers (past 48hrs)

Breakfast, lunch, dinner, supper, snacks and water intake (past 48hrs)

Notes

Migraine Event Tracker

Date: Day | Mon   Tue   Wed   Thu   Fri   Sat   Sun

Time started: Duration (hr/min):   Severity (1-9):

Time ended: Sleep (hr/min):

Symptoms experienced

Activities and possible triggers (past 48hrs)

Breakfast, lunch, dinner, supper, snacks and water intake (past 48hrs)

Notes

Migraine Event Tracker

Date: Day | Mon   Tue   Wed   Thu   Fri   Sat   Sun

Time started: Duration (hr/min):   Severity (1-9):

Time ended: Sleep (hr/min):

Symptoms experienced

Activities and possible triggers (past 48hrs)

Breakfast, lunch, dinner, supper, snacks and water intake (past 48hrs)

Notes

Migraine Event Tracker

Date: _____   Day | Mon   Tue   Wed   Thu   Fri   Sat   Sun

Time started: _____   Duration (hr/min): _____   Severity (1-9): _____

Time ended: _____   Sleep (hr/min): _____

Symptoms experienced

Activities and possible triggers (past 48hrs)

Breakfast, lunch, dinner, supper, snacks and water intake (past 48hrs)

Notes

Migraine Event Tracker

Date: Day | Mon   Tue   Wed   Thu   Fri   Sat   Sun

Time started: Duration (hr/min):   Severity (1-9):

Time ended: Sleep (hr/min):

Symptoms experienced

Activities and possible triggers (past 48hrs)

Breakfast, lunch, dinner, supper, snacks and water intake (past 48hrs)

Notes

Migraine Event Tracker

Date: _____ Day | Mon Tue Wed Thu Fri Sat Sun

Time started: _____ Duration (hr/min): _____ Severity (1-9): _____

Time ended: _____ Sleep (hr/min): _____

Symptoms experienced

Activities and possible triggers (past 48hrs)

Breakfast, lunch, dinner, supper, snacks and water intake (past 48hrs)

Notes

Migraine Event Tracker

Date: Day | Mon   Tue   Wed   Thu   Fri   Sat   Sun

Time started: Duration (hr/min):   Severity (1-9):

Time ended: Sleep (hr/min):

Symptoms experienced

Activities and possible triggers (past 48hrs)

Breakfast, lunch, dinner, supper, snacks and water intake (past 48hrs)

Notes

Migraine Event Tracker

Date: Day | Mon   Tue   Wed   Thu   Fri   Sat   Sun

Time started: Duration (hr/min):   Severity (1-9):

Time ended: Sleep (hr/min):

Symptoms experienced

Activities and possible triggers (past 48hrs)

Breakfast, lunch, dinner, supper, snacks and water intake (past 48hrs)

Notes

Migraine Event Tracker

Date: Day | Mon   Tue   Wed   Thu   Fri   Sat   Sun

Time started: Duration (hr/min):   Severity (1-9):

Time ended: Sleep (hr/min):

Symptoms experienced

Activities and possible triggers (past 48hrs)

Breakfast, lunch, dinner, supper, snacks and water intake (past 48hrs)

Notes

Migraine Event Tracker

Date: _____ Day | Mon Tue Wed Thu Fri Sat Sun

Time started: _____ Duration (hr/min): _____ Severity (1-9): _____

Time ended: _____ Sleep (hr/min): _____

Symptoms experienced

Activities and possible triggers (past 48hrs)

Breakfast, lunch, dinner, supper, snacks and water intake (past 48hrs)

Notes

Migraine Event Tracker

Date: Day | Mon   Tue   Wed   Thu   Fri   Sat   Sun

Time started: Duration (hr/min):   Severity (1-9):

Time ended: Sleep (hr/min):

Symptoms experienced

Activities and possible triggers (past 48hrs)

Breakfast, lunch, dinner, supper, snacks and water intake (past 48hrs)

Notes

Migraine Event Tracker

Date: Day | Mon   Tue   Wed   Thu   Fri   Sat   Sun

Time started: Duration (hr/min):   Severity (1-9):

Time ended: Sleep (hr/min):

Symptoms experienced

Activities and possible triggers (past 48hrs)

Breakfast, lunch, dinner, supper, snacks and water intake (past 48hrs)

Notes

Migraine Event Tracker

Date: Day | Mon   Tue   Wed   Thu   Fri   Sat   Sun

Time started: Duration (hr/min):   Severity (1-9):

Time ended: Sleep (hr/min):

Symptoms experienced

Activities and possible triggers (past 48hrs)

Breakfast, lunch, dinner, supper, snacks and water intake (past 48hrs)

Notes

Migraine Event Tracker

Date: Day | Mon   Tue   Wed   Thu   Fri   Sat   Sun

Time started: Duration (hr/min):   Severity (1-9):

Time ended: Sleep (hr/min):

Symptoms experienced

Activities and possible triggers (past 48hrs)

Breakfast, lunch, dinner, supper, snacks and water intake (past 48hrs)

Notes

Migraine Event Tracker

Date: _____   Day | Mon   Tue   Wed   Thu   Fri   Sat   Sun

Time started: _____   Duration (hr/min): _____   Severity (1-9): _____

Time ended: _____   Sleep (hr/min): _____

Symptoms experienced

Activities and possible triggers (past 48hrs)

Breakfast, lunch, dinner, supper, snacks and water intake (past 48hrs)

Notes

Migraine Event Tracker

Date: Day | Mon   Tue   Wed   Thu   Fri   Sat   Sun

Time started: Duration (hr/min):   Severity (1-9):

Time ended: Sleep (hr/min):

Symptoms experienced

Activities and possible triggers (past 48hrs)

Breakfast, lunch, dinner, supper, snacks and water intake (past 48hrs)

Notes

Migraine Event Tracker

Date: Day | Mon   Tue   Wed   Thu   Fri   Sat   Sun

Time started: Duration (hr/min):   Severity (1-9):

Time ended: Sleep (hr/min):

Symptoms experienced

Activities and possible triggers (past 48hrs)

Breakfast, lunch, dinner, supper, snacks and water intake (past 48hrs)

Notes

Migraine Event Tracker

Date: Day | Mon Tue Wed Thu Fri Sat Sun

Time started: Duration (hr/min): Severity (1-9):

Time ended: Sleep (hr/min):

Symptoms experienced

Activities and possible triggers (past 48hrs)

Breakfast, lunch, dinner, supper, snacks and water intake (past 48hrs)

Notes

Migraine Event Tracker

Date: _____ Day | Mon Tue Wed Thu Fri Sat Sun

Time started: _____ Duration (hr/min): _____ Severity (1-9): _____

Time ended: _____ Sleep (hr/min): _____

Symptoms experienced

Activities and possible triggers (past 48hrs)

Breakfast, lunch, dinner, supper, snacks and water intake (past 48hrs)

Notes

Migraine Event Tracker

Date: Day | Mon   Tue   Wed   Thu   Fri   Sat   Sun

Time started: Duration (hr/min):   Severity (1-9):

Time ended: Sleep (hr/min):

Symptoms experienced

Activities and possible triggers (past 48hrs)

Breakfast, lunch, dinner, supper, snacks and water intake (past 48hrs)

Notes

Notes |

Notes |